Summary of

The Sleep Revolution

Transforming Your Life, One Night at a Time

by Arianna Huffington

Instaread

Please Note

This is a summary with analysis.

Table of Contents

Overview

The Sleep Revolution is a call to action to make sleep a priority and reclaim the night for the basic human need of rest. Millions of people use nighttime hours for activities other than sleep. They choose to prioritize work or succumb to an addiction to technology rather than invest those precious hours in sleep. In the United States and increasingly around the world, work culture regards sleep as an inefficient waste of time.

However, getting enough sleep can be a matter of life or death. People who have deprived themselves of sleep have, in some cases, collapsed or even died. Others have suffered and ended up in the hospital due to dangerous levels of exhaustion. Even less extreme sleep deprivation has resulted in physical and mental damage.

Throughout history, many different cultures have held a profound appreciation of sleep. The ancient Greeks and Egyptians would sleep in temples to have their dreams interpreted by priests. They believed that time at rest offered a sacred connection to the gods. In the Bible,

Joseph rose to prominence by demonstrating his ability to interpret the dreams of the Pharaoh. Centuries later, but before the invention of the lightbulb and the rise of industrialization, people would go to bed when the sun went down. With so many long hours in darkness, people tended to experience a bifurcated sleep in which a period of wakefulness could be spent in quiet meditation or engaging in other tasks before returning to rest. In this split sleeping time, the waking portion of the night was a time to be enjoyed or utilized. In modern times, by contrast, being awake in the middle of the night is a potential source of great anxiety.

Keeping smartphones within arm's reach of the bed— even on our pillows—damages our relation to sleep. Tools for assisting sleep and remaining awake have only made things worse. Many people drink excessive caffeine by day and then use sleeping pills to power down at night.

The relationship to sleep in the modern industrialized world is troubled, but the problem is not intractable. Daytime naps can prove restorative and can help undo the damage of a sleepless night. Meditation and a healthy lifestyle that includes exercise can help people make it through the night without the assistance of medication. While some solutions may work for certain people and not others, it's vital to find one that works for any given individual because as sleep habits affect every aspect of human life.

Important People

Arianna Huffington is the co-founder and editor-in-chief of *The Huffington Post*. She is the author of 15 books on a wide range of topics including a biography of Pablo Picasso and an illustrated guide to the gods of her native Greece. She has been named as one of the most powerful women in the world today. [1]

Key Takeaways

1. Sleep is a basic human need that is vital to our survival.

2. Around the world, the human relationship to sleep is in crisis.

3. Getting a full night's sleep has never been harder to achieve.

4. Cultural values that promote a lack of sleep as a means to achieve success are the root cause of the contemporary sleep deprivation crisis.

5. Recent advancements in sleep science are providing the evidence needed to overturn the culture of sleep deprivation.

6. Sleep deprivation does not impact every race, economic class, and gender equally.

7. Lack of sleep has very real financial and human costs.

8. The tools we currently use to assist our sleep-deprived lifestyle do more harm than good.

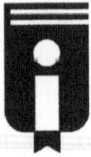

Thank you for purchasing this Instaread book

Download the Instaread mobile app to get
unlimited text & audio summaries
of bestselling books.

Visit Instaread.co
to learn more.

Analysis

Key Takeaway 1

Sleep is a basic human need that is vital to our survival.

Analysis

Sleep is essential to every part of our lives. It impacts our health, our happiness, and our abilities to work and function. While we sleep, the body—in particular the brain—is performing necessary functions to protect our memories and our sanity.

Sleep is such an important component of the human ability to survive that sleep deprivation has often been employed as a means of torture. In the prison at Guantánamo Bay, Cuba, sleep deprivation has been used as a means of "enhanced interrogation." [2] The United Nations Committee Against Torture has called on the United States to abolish the use of sleep deprivation on prisoners. [3] Within as little as a day, people who are sleep deprived could begin to suffer from psychosis. [4]

Sleep is crucial in the healing process. However, the noise level in many hospitals makes it very difficult for patients to get adequate sleep. In a 2013 article for *The Atlantic*, physician Peter Ubel recounted his own visit to the hospital for surgery on a kidney tumor. While his procedure went without complications, he found it impossible to sleep afterwards because frequent checks of his vital signs and overnight blood draws awoke him repeatedly. The beeping of his IV machine would wake him intermittently as well. As a result, he found that not an hour of sleep was allowed to progress uninterrupted at a time when sleep could not possibly have been more important to his well-being. Ubel recommends changes in hospital protocol that would consolidate many interruptions into just one or two by having staff perform more than one test or vital check at a time. This, he argues, would dramatically improve patient outcomes and assist in the healing process. [5]

Key Takeaway 2

Around the world, the human relationship to sleep is in crisis.

Analysis

The average adult should be getting seven hours of sleep every night. However, more than 40 percent of Americans are not. Global statistics are similar, if not more alarming.

Many people take action to curb risky behaviors, such as smoking or drinking alcohol to excess, with the hopes of leading a healthier life. Yet they don't think twice about scrimping on hours of sleep when a seemingly more important task for work arises. However, Oxford neuroscientist Dr. Russell Foster is reframing exactly how dangerous it is to skip on sleep. He has suggested that sleeping less than five hours per day carries health consequences that are comparable to those sustained by smoking. Foster said that lack of sleep impairs function enough to make sleepy subjects behave similar to the way they would if they were drunk. [6]

Key Takeaway 3

Getting a full night's sleep has never been harder to achieve.

Analysis

Technology has irrevocably changed the human relationship to sleep. Cell phones and other devices are typically blamed for this shift. When their circadian rhythm is disrupted by caffeine or erratic sleep patterns, many people turn to a device when unable to sleep. In 2015, more than 70 percent of Americans kept their cellphones either in their beds or directly next to them. Dependence on these devices for distraction inhibits the peace of mind required to fall asleep. Devices can also disrupt a sleeping person if they are not silenced, and increased dependence on devices drives users deeper into a cycle of sleeplessness.

However, even the humble lightbulb has forever changed the ways in which we choose when to go to bed instead of letting the sun decide for us. In the 150 years since the advent of the lightbulb, humans have been able to extend the workday without regard to natural diurnal patterns of light and dark. As a result, work and technological entertainment compete as never before with sleep for our time and attention.

Key Takeaway 4

Cultural values that promote a lack of sleep as a means to achieve success are the root cause of the contemporary sleep deprivation crisis.

Analysis

In centuries past, sleep was understood to be sacred—both literally as a means of communicating with a higher power and figuratively as a vital part of life not to be disrupted. However, sleep is no longer prioritized in this way. In many contexts, people associate sleep with a waste of time and brag about their lack of time spent in bed as a way of communicating their drive for success. To actually bring about a change in the sleep crisis, we must adjust our cultural outlook on sleep.

A culture that rewards lack of sleep as a sign of dedication to work is one that is rooted in arrogance, according to University of Oxford Professor Russell Foster. He slams the braggadocio surrounding middle-of-the-night emails and world leaders' claims of little sleep while on the job as tantamount to believing "we can abandon four billion years of evolution and ignore the fact that we have evolved under a light-dark cycle." [7] The belief that those who can defeat the natural human instinct for sleep are stronger or more poised for success is, from Foster's perspective, inherently false.

Sleep habits have worsened in recent decades with most Americans seeing increasingly demanding work schedules. People today get, on average, two hours of sleep less than their counterparts did in the 1950s. [8] With so many ways to communicate today—email, for one—those middle-of-the night time stamps send a message of their own beyond whatever may be actually included in the communication. The senders hope it will be perceived by superiors and peers as a sign of commitment and ambition. However, by rewarding this effort, people are ultimately failing their health and their bodies—both of which require sleep. Randi Zuckerberg, entrepreneur and social media maven, recommends that companies shut off their internal email services from 9 p.m. until the following morning so that no one can be specifically praised for working through the night. [9]

Key Takeaway 5

Recent advancements in sleep science are providing the evidence needed to overturn the culture of sleep deprivation.

Analysis

There are more scientists researching sleep than ever before. This new focus on the importance of sleep is helping the scientific community communicate to laypersons that it's time to upend the crisis of chronic sleep deprivation and reclaim control over this vital process. It is more possible than ever to research our personal sleeping habits with the advent of sleep trackers and other wearable technology that provide data and insights into the quality and quantity of our sleep.

Recent studies have furthered our understanding of why we sleep by night and are awake during the day. Studying plankton, researchers found that the role of the brain chemical melatonin—which is responsible for our circadian cycles—first evolved in our microscopic, underwater ancestors some 700 million years ago. A German study was then able to link the genes of a small ocean worm to our own and found that the worm, much like us, only produces melatonin at night. The similarities were so strong that researchers were able to simulate jet lag in these worms by exposing them to darkness when their body clocks were predicting daylight. [10] By understanding that the need to sleep is wired into our evolution and our genetic code, perhaps people can begin to learn that trying to defeat the nightly urge to rest is to deny hundreds of millions of years of progress.

Sleep trackers can help people understand the importance of getting a full night's rest. Fitbit, for example, provides its users with a very thorough picture of their night's activity. The wearable device does not merely measure whether or not the user slept. It provides data on when the user was sleeping heavily and for how long. It also notes periods of restlessness. With a little bit of homework, a user can get a better picture of the impact of sleep on daily life. [11] For example, a man may find that on a night when he slept only four hours, he logged 1,000 additional calories in the food tracking side of the app. Or he may notice that his workout, which he tracked in the app, was very much less robust than average. Seeing this personalized data—even if imperfect—can give him a broad overview of how sleep impacts his life and compel him to take more control over his nighttime activities.

Key Takeaway 6

Sleep deprivation does not impact every race, economic class, and gender equally.

Analysis

Sleep deprivation is not universally a problem of equal scale. A University of Chicago study found that people living in communities of lower socioeconomic status experience poorer sleep quality than their wealthier counterparts. Regardless of income, women tend to bear the brunt of sleep deprivation in their households more than their male counterparts. As women tend to carry the weight of childcare and home chores in addition to their day jobs, many women find it harder to get the rest they need than the men in their households.

While the sleep quality found in lower socioeconomic areas may be poor, the Centers for Disease Control and Prevention found that Americans living below the poverty line were the most likely to get the most sleep, nine hours or more. However, when these figures are broken down by race, it becomes clear that there are major differences in how much we sleep. More than 34 percent of black adults sleep six hours or less in a given night, making them more likely to be sleep deprived than their white or Asian counterparts. The CDC found that divorced or separated adults were most likely to sleep less than six hours—much more so than people who are married, were never married, or who cohabit. When the figures are broken down geographically, adults living in the western states are the most likely to get the recommended seven to eight hours of sleep. People living in the Northeast were the least likely to sleep the recommended number of hours. [12]

Key Takeaway 7

Lack of sleep has very real financial and human costs.

Analysis

Every year, lack of sleep costs businesses an average of 11 days of work per employee. The associated health costs can be enormous. Sleep-deprived workers cost employers about $2,280 per employee and the national economy more than $63 billion in a single year.

Nurses logging their sleep and workplace errors noted 3.3 times as many medical errors when their shifts ran 12.5 hours instead of 8.5 hours. [13] Similarly, interns who often worked long night shifts in intensive-care units made five times as many diagnostic errors than their counterparts with shorter shifts. [14] This data makes it clear that the human and financial costs of sleep deprivation can be staggering.

Key Takeaway 8

The tools we currently use to assist our sleep-deprived lifestyle do more harm than good.

Analysis

Because of our chronic state of sleep deprivation, Americans are relying increasingly on sleeping pills to fall asleep. In the morning, an alarm clock heralds the start to many of our days by shocking us into wakefulness with a jolt of adrenaline. From there, we continue to ramp up the cycle of stimulation throughout the day with increasingly large doses of caffeine. When night comes, many of us succumb to sleeping pills or an alcoholic beverage—both of which fail to provide the same quality of sleep that would come to us naturally. Rather than pursue artificial solutions, we should seek natural sleep by cutting our reliance on caffeine and make up for lost nighttime sleep hours with a nap during the day.

In a survey from 2013, researchers learned that 1 in 20 teens went to school in the morning after having substituted breakfast with a high-caffeine energy drink. [15] Recognizing this trend in their own students, Haydock High School in England banned energy drinks including Red Bull, Monster, and any other enhanced-caffeine beverage. Within two semesters of creating this policy in 2014, the school's principal reported that detentions had dropped by a third and that teachers had observed a marked improvement in student performance. [16]

The results suggested that cutting off artificial stimulants in school and thereby encouraging students to come to school rested was responsible for the decline in behavioral problems.

Author's Style

Arianna Huffington combines personal perspective with research and analysis to build a compelling argument for why sleep matters to our health, happiness, and livelihoods. Although her research is thorough, she does, at times, make correlations that the studies she cites do not necessarily support. For example, she concludes without real evidence that famously sleep-deprived former President Bill Clinton may have made poor decisions on gays in the military while in office because he was not getting his needed rest.

Part analysis, part self-help book, *The Sleep Revolution* provides the reader with many of Huffington's favorite strategies for getting good rest and includes several supplements at the end of her text to teach the reader self-guided meditation techniques. Huffington punctuates her chapters with the inclusion of short passages or poems about sleep from renowned authors.

Author's Perspective

Huffington grew up in a tiny one-bedroom apartment in Greece where her mother taught her and her siblings that sleep was sacred and not to be interrupted. But in later years, she learned to neglect these valuable lessons. As the co-founder and editor-in-chief of *The Huffington Post* and a sought-after media personality, Huffington spends much of her life traveling or working. In 2007, she found herself struggling to balance her professional life and her family time with her two daughters. On one of her daughter's tours to select a university, Huffington began working through the night. She believed that she could be fully present by day on the college visits and still work several hours after her daughter went to bed. Ultimately, she collapsed from sleep exhaustion in 2007. This moment alerted Huffington that she needed to make serious changes. She became protective of her sleep habits and even gained notoriety for installing private napping pods in her company's newsroom. She chose to write *The Sleep Revolution* as part of an effort to change prevailing attitudes toward sleep.

~~~~ END OF INSTAREAD ~~~~

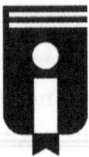

Thank you for purchasing this Instaread book

**Download the Instaread mobile app to get
unlimited text & audio summaries
of bestselling books.**

Visit Instaread.co
to learn more.

References

1. "The World's 100 Most Powerful Women (2015)." *Forbes.* Accessed April 14, 2016. http://www.forbes.com/power-women/list/2/#tab:overall

2. Laughland, Oliver. "How the CIA tortured its detainees." *The Guardian,* May 20, 2015. Accessed May 5, 2016. http://www.theguardian.com/us-news/2014/dec/09/cia-torture-methods-waterboarding-sleep-deprivation

3. Human Rights Watch. "Submission to the United Nations Committee against Torture." March 1, 2016. Accessed April 14, 2016. https://www.hrw.org/news/2016/03/01/submission-united-nations-committee-against-torture

4. Petrovsky, Nadine, et al. "Sleep Deprivation Disrupts Prepulse Inhibition and Induces Psychosis-Like Symptoms in Healthy Humans." *Journal of Neuroscience* 34:27 (July 2, 2014): 9134-140. Accessed April 14, 2016. http://www.jneurosci.org/content/34/27/9134.short

5. Ubel, Peter. "Sleep Deprivation in Hospitals Is a Real Problem." *The Atlantic,* June 19, 2013. Accessed April 14, 2016. http://www.theatlantic.com/health/archive/2013/06/sleep-deprivation-in-hospitals-is-a-real-problem/276960/

6. Donnelly, Laura. "Sleep deprivation 'as bad as smoking.'" *The Telegraph,* July 27, 2015. Accessed

April 14, 2016. http://www.telegraph.co.uk/news/health/11765723/Sleep-deprivation-as-bad-as-smoking.html

7. Gallagher, James. "'Arrogance' of Ignoring Need for Sleep." BBC News, May 12, 2014. Accessed April 14, 2016. http://www.bbc.com/news/health-27286872

8. Rock, Lucy. "It's time to stop this competitive sleep deprivation." *The Guardian*, May 16, 2014. Accessed April 14, 2016. http://www.theguardian.com/theobserver/she-said/2014/may/16/its-time-to-stop-this-competitive-sleep-deprivation

9. Zuckerberg, Randi. "The 2 A.M. Email: A Public Display Of Ambition." *LinkedIn Pulse*, April 23, 2013. Accessed April 14, 2016. https://www.linkedin.com/pulse/20130423140003-8628736-the-2-a-m-email-a-public-display-of-ambition.

10. Tosches, Maria Antonietta, et al. "Melatonin Signaling Controls Circadian Swimming Behavior in Marine Zooplankton." *Cell* 159, no. 1 (September 2014): 46-57. Accessed April 14, 2016. http://www.ncbi.nlm.nih.gov/pmc/articles/PMC4182423/

11. Stables, James. "Fitbit to 'vigorously defend' its sleep tracking tech in 'meritless' lawsuit." *Wareable*, May 13, 2015. Accessed April 14, 2016. http://www.wareable.com/fitbit/fitbit-targeted-in-sleep-tracking-lawsuit-1133

12. Schoenborn, C.A. and P.F. Adams. "Health Behaviors of Adults: United States, 2005–2007." Vital and Health Statistics, 10:245 (March 2010). Accessed April 14, 2016. http://www.cdc.gov/nchs/data/series/sr_10/sr10_245.pdf

13. Scott, Linda D., et al. "The Relationship between Nurse Work Schedules, Sleep Duration, and Drowsy Driving." *Sleep.* 30:12 (December 2007):1801-1807. Accessed May 4, 2016. http://www.ncbi.nlm.nih.gov/pmc/articles/PMC2276124/

14. Landrigan, CP, et al. "Effect of reducing interns' work hours on serious medical errors in intensive care units." *New England Journal of Medicine.* 2004; 351(18):1838-48. Accessed May 4, 2016. http://www.ncbi.nlm.nih.gov/pubmed/15509817

15. Tozer, James. "School that banned Red Bull sees detention plunge by a third." *The Daily Mail,* December 4, 2014. Accessed April 14, 2016. http://www.dailymail.co.uk/news/article-2861039/School-slashes-number-detentions-issued-banning-energy-drinks.html

16. Jeffay, John. "School BANS Red Bull and the number of detentions falls, claims headteacher." *The Mirror,* December 4, 2014. Accessed April 14, 2016. http://www.mirror.co.uk/news/uk-news/school-bans-red-bull-number-4750944

Lightning Source UK Ltd.
Milton Keynes UK
UKOW06f2351170816

280960UK00021B/528/P